Ketogenic Diet

Ketogenic diet for beginners including recipes, ketosis for weight loss, what ketosis is, and more!

Table of Contents

Introduction

Thank you for taking the time to pick up this book on the ketogenic diet!

This book covers the topic of ketogenic diets and will teach you all about ketosis and its health benefits!

Ketogenic diets have been used for thousands of years for their many health benefits, ease of implementation, and simply because of the environments we evolved in. Soon, you will discover all about the ketogenic diet, how ketosis works, and why exactly you shouldn't fear eating fat like the media often tells us to!

At the completion of this book you will have a good understanding of the ketogenic diet, its benefits, and know exactly how to begin living a ketogenic lifestyle.

This book contains tips for making the transition into a ketogenic lifestyle a smooth one, and even provides some recipes to help you to dive right in!

Once again, thanks for taking the time to read this book, I hope you find it to be helpful, and wish you the best of luck in your journey towards becoming a better, healthier, and more energetic you!

Chapter 1:
What is a Ketogenic Diet?

The ketogenic diet has often been regarded as a fad that is sure to fade with time. However, some form of the ketogenic diet has always existed, and is still being implicated by celebrities, fitness gurus, and even holistic doctors for its miraculous benefits and overall rate of success. You may have heard the keto diet called the "low carb," "high fat, low carb," or "Atkins" diet. Although many have heard of the ketogenic lifestyle, very few actually understand the structure of the program and the life-changing effects it can have.

Many diets require the user to take supplements, or add or take away something from an organized meal plan. A ketogenic lifestyle has its own limitations, but the entire process is completely natural. One of the key points of going ketogenic is cutting out all of the processed sugar, preservatives, and chemicals that are regularly added to food products, and allowing your body to function off of natural, organic, *real* food. The reality is that our bodies were not meant to consume heavy sugars, simple carbohydrates, gluten, or GMO's. Allowing your body to detox and heal from the influence of these ingredients will not only promote drastic weight loss, but also will result in increased energy, a healthy immune system, and overall health and wellbeing.

What is a Ketogenic Diet?

A ketogenic diet is when an individual limits their meals to whole, natural foods that are low in sugar; while also increasing their fat and protein intake. It is considered to be 'ketogenic' when your body enters a state known as 'ketosis' which occurs when you consume a very low amount of carbohydrates.

As previously mentioned, you may have heard of a "low carb, no carb" diet. A ketogenic diet is essentially cutting carbohydrates from your diet and essentially eating just meat, vegetables, and a few other chosen foods.

Sugar comes in various forms: glucose, fructose, sucrose, and carbohydrates. You may have heard that it is better to snack on fruit than a candy bar; however, a large banana has roughly the same amount of sugar as a bottle of soda. In other words, when it comes to the ketogenic diet, sugar is sugar regardless of what form it comes in. It doesn't matter if you are eating "healthy" sugar (fructose), or processed sugars, it will have a similar effect on your body and keep you from going into ketosis. Before you can understand how your body works in a ketogenic state, you must know how your body processes sugar.

When you consume food that is high in carbohydrates, your body produces glucose and insulin. Glucose is the easiest form of sugar that your body can break down to use for energy. When you eat or drink anything, your body will first use the glucose, which is why you get a sudden burst of energy when you eat a meal that has a significant number of carbs. Your body produces insulin in response to the glucose in your bloodstream because too much glucose in your bloodstream can be deadly, and insulin naturally brings those blood sugar levels down. The excess sugar and fat that is not used right away as energy is stored away for later. This is your body's natural response to a potential threat of famine. Our ancestors experience famine and disease much more than we do now, and their struggles have led our bodies to become evolved in anticipation of such an occurrence. That is why, when you eat at a calorie deficit, your body uses stored fat for energy and survival, and you lose weight.

This is essentially what a ketogenic diet does; it is lowering your intake of carbs so that your body can go into survival mode and convert stored fat for energy. This state is called ketosis. During ketosis, your body produces ketones, which are created from the fats that are broken down in the liver. The primary goal of a ketogenic diet is to make your body go into this metabolic state in order to gain certain health benefits, as well as to shape and sculpt your body.

Eliminating carbs form your diet does not mean that you are starving yourself of calories, but of sugar. During a ketogenic diet, you are still able to eat at a caloric maintenance or even a caloric surplus. To do this, you must force your body to use fat as its main source of energy instead of carbohydrates.

What Do I Eat on a Ketogenic Diet?

A true ketogenic diet usually requires a lot of planning ahead, by meal prepping and having a practical meal plan already in place. Your meal plan wholly depends on how fast you want to enter a ketogenic state; the more restrictive you are with carbohydrates the faster ketosis will happen. If you want to ease your way into strategically cutting back on carbs, then it will take longer to get into ketosis.

If you take a look at any standard food label, you will see a detailed breakdown of all of the nutrients and ingredients that are in each serving. While you may be used to counting calories, you are now counting carbs and will have to pay attention to how many grams of carbohydrates are in each serving and in the entire product. You will also notice that every food label breaks down carbohydrates into total carbs, dietary fiber, and sugar. While the key is to avoid all carbs when on a ketogenic diet, many foods have fiber; in which case you will have to simply count the net carbs instead. A net carb is the total dietary carbohydrates in a food product, minus the amount of fiber.

Learning Your Macros

It is nearly impossible to eliminate all carbs from your diet, as even vegetables have sugar in them! However, as long as you stay on track with your carb intake, you can easily experience the full benefits of ketosis. Your nutrient intake is the most important factor of ketogenic and weight loss success. Therefore, you need to break down your meal plans and daily meal regiments into specific macro percentages. Your total nutrient intake should be approximately seventy percent fats, twenty- five percent protein, and five percent carb. The set number of grams for each nutrient category is determined based on your goals, current weight, activity level, etc. You can easily find a calculator online that will help you determine how much of each nutrient you should consume. However, it is standard that you should consume less than thirty grams of carbohydrates a day in order to enter ketosis, and less than fifteen grams per day if you'd like to enter ketosis rapidly. The lower that you keep your glucose levels, the better your results will be.

The carbohydrates that you do eat should come in the form of vegetables, nuts, and some dairy products. Many ketogenic dieters keep cheese, butter, plain yogurt, and sour cream in their diets to enhance the flavors of their food. You want to stay away from all refined sugars, such as wheat products, starch, and fruit. This may seem incredibly difficult, but the results are absolutely worth the sacrifice. There are thousands of recipes that will keep your sugar cravings at bay and help your body easily adjust to your new lifestyle. Most of your meals should be protein, with a side of vegetables, and an extra serving of fat.

One of the most common myths in the diet and health industry is that fat is bad for your body, and will make you fat. However, fat does *not* make you fat. In fact, consuming a high fat, low carb diet will help to cleanse your organs and shed stubborn fat. It is simply the combination of fat with sugar that results in weight gain. The following food list will help to guide you as you begin your ketogenic journey.

Ketogenic Grocery List

<u>**Meat**</u>

Beef

Chicken

Fish

Turkey

Pork

Eggs

<u>**Vegetables**</u>- Some vegetables have more carbs than others. For example, broccoli may have four grams of carbs per cup, but a tomato has more. For the first two months or so of your ketogenic diet, you should stick to this list of vegetables before introducing the veggies that are missing back into your meal plan.

Artichoke

Arugula

Asparagus

Alfalfa Sprouts

Bok Choy

Broccoli

Brussel Sprouts

Cabbage

Cauliflower

Celery

Chard

Collard Greens

Eggplant

Fennel

Garlic

Green Beans

Herbs

Kale

Leek

Lettuce

Mushrooms

Onions

Shallot

Spinach

Parsley

Bell Peppers

Chili Peppers

Zucchini

Fats

Avocado Oil

Canola Oil

Coconut Oil

Flaxseed Oil

Grapeseed Oil

Hemp Seed Oil

Olive Oil

Sesame Oil

Sunflower Oil

Vegetable Oil

<u>Dairy</u>- It is crucial that you limit your dairy intake, as it can lead to excess water weight, or consuming more carbs than your plan permits. Most dairy products do have some sugar; so consuming them in moderation will keep your taste buds happy while still allowing you to maintain your ketogenic state.

Butter

Cheese

Cream Cheese

Milk – It can have a significant amount of added sugar, so you should opt for half and half for your morning coffee or tea instead of your usual creamer.

Heavy Whipping Cream - Heavy whipping cream has a lot of fat in it, which will make it a little bit easier for you to reach your daily fat intake. However, heavy cream is high in calories, so be careful with your portion sizes.

<u>Nuts and Seeds</u>

Almonds

Cashews

Chestnuts

Hazelnuts

Macadamia

Peanuts

Pecans

Pine Nuts

Pistachio

Walnuts

Chia Seeds

Hemp Seeds

Flaxseeds

Pumpkin Seeds

Sesame Seeds

Sunflower Seeds

Beverages

Water (Plain or Sparkling)

Tea (No Added Sugar)

Coffee (No Added Sugar)

Off Limit Foods

Dairy

Buttermilk

Butterfat

Custard

Milk

Ice Cream

Yogurt

<u>Vegetables</u>

Beans

Carrots

Corn

Chickpeas

Hummus

Lentils

Parsnip

Peas

Tomatoes

<u>Starches</u>

Potatoes

Pumpkin

Sweet Potatoes

Squash

Rice

<u>Grains</u>

Bread

Bagels

Curry

Couscous

English Muffins

Pasta

Rolls

Tortillas

Whole Grains

<u>All Fruits</u>

<u>All Dessert Foods</u>

<u>Tomato- Based Products</u>

Ketchup

Tomato Sauce

Tomato Paste

<u>Miscellaneous Foods</u>

Nuts Butters

Candy Products

Chips

Gravy

Jellies and Preserves

Pretzels

Soups and Broths

Popcorn

Soy Products

Syrups

<u>Anything Labeled "Fat Free"</u>

Sugar and Artificial Sweeteners

White Sugar

Brown Sugar

Cane Sugar

Powdered Sugar

Aspartame

Agave Nectar

Erythritol

Sucralose

Stevia

Xylitol

Beverages

Juice

Soda

Kool- Aid

Tang

Sports Drinks

Energy Drinks

Sweetened Tea

Sweetened Coffee Products

Milk

Hot Chocolate

All Alcoholic Beverages

Chapter 2:
Your Body During Ketosis

Your body normally converts glucose into energy, which is why you may feel a burst of energy after a big meal. Over time, your body creates enzymes ready to aid this process, with only a few enzymes prepared to handle fats, mostly to store the fat molecules. However, while on a ketogenic diet, your body uses protein and fat for energy instead so that you don't have to rely on sugar to keep you going throughout the day.

Now that you increased your intake of fats, your body suddenly has to build up a new store of enzymes to aid the breakdown process. During the beginning of entering a ketogenic state, your body will use up the last stores of glucose before using fat for energy. This will deplete all glycogen from your muscles, resulting in a temporary lack of energy and lethargy. Your body is essentially detoxing from sugar, resulting in a number of withdrawal symptoms. Sugar is ten times more addictive than cocaine, and is the most used "drug" in the world. When you do not feed into sugar cravings, your body will initially react negatively. Some of the most common symptoms that you may experience include:

- Headaches

- Gas and Bloating

- Mental Fogginess

- Lethargy

- Insomnia

- Dizziness

- Irritability and Mood Swings

- Nausea

- Achiness

Many of the symptoms are also in response to the electrolytes that your body will be flushing out, as a ketogenic state has a diuretic effect. If you start to experience any of these symptoms, you must resist the urge to give into your addiction and consume sugar. Instead, drink plenty of water and increase your sodium intake. This will not only help balance your electrolytes, but will also aid with water retention for a flatter stomach.

For individuals who go to the gym on a regular basis, it is especially crucial that you stay on track with your ketogenic diet and increase your water intake. Your diet makes up eighty percent of your weight loss success, and the leftover twenty is the result of your active time at the gym. This means that keeping up this strict ketogenic diet is more important right now than going to the gym and trying to burn a few extra calories. Regardless, the sudden lack of carbohydrates will lead to a drop in your energy level and contribute to a drastic change in your mood and productivity. This is completely normal, but you may feel guilty about choosing to sit on the couch watching television over going to the gym. In this case, it is best if you *do* rest instead of doing physical activity, so that you do not expend all of your energy at the gym and end up feeling worse after a workout.

How Do I Lose Fat by Eating Fat?

Fat has been demonized by the food and health industry for decades. The pharmaceutical industry makes billions of dollars from conditions and diseases that are the result of high sugar intake, with the food industry following suit with fat-free foods. Why would modern health professionals encourage you to cut out carbs when many people are willing to pay extra for special food and magic pills that are especially made for individuals who want to lose weight, control their type two diabetes, and prevent heart disease? Eating processed sugars and refined carbs leads to a number of severe health problems that have been linked to the development of diabetes, cancer, and obesity. Everyone wants to know the secret to burning fat, losing weight, being healthy, etc.; when the answer is simple: cut out carbs and eat fat.

The misunderstanding that fat makes you fat comes from the knowledge that fat has more calories than carbs do. And since the diet and weight loss industry thrives on counting calories rather than your sugar intake, it makes sense to cut calories by cutting out fat from your diet. The bodybuilding community knows better than anyone that to efficiently cut down their body fat percentage and create a sculptured body they must stop eating carbs and increase their dietary fat intake. This is because low-fat diets do not condition your body to efficiently burn fat, but actually help it become better are converting sugar into energy. Low-fat diets also lower the amount of adipokines (a fat burning hormone) in your body, which will slow your metabolism and increase your appetite.

So how does your body make protein and fat turn into energy?

Protein

The protein you eat is broken down in to amino acids, which are used to build muscle, restore damaged muscles, aid protein-based hormone production, transport molecules throughout your body, and creates antibodies – which help fight disease and illness. Your body can convert protein into energy, but sometimes it comes at a price. If you consume too much protein, it will be converted into glucose, then stored as fat for later. This will knock you out of ketosis and you will have to start the process of entering a ketogenic state all over again.

Fat

Fats usually provide your body with more than half of its energy needs. When fat is transported through your digestive tract and into the small intestine, cholestokinin (a hormone) signals your gallbladder to release bile. Bile allows fat to combine with water so that lipase can break down the fat into fatty acids and glycerol. Lipase is an enzyme that breaks down fats you consume so that the intestines can break them down. Lipase is created in your mouth, stomach, and pancreas. The small molecules are either stored in fat cells in body tissue that store fat, or are absorbed by cells in the intestinal wall.

Within the intestinal wall, the broken down fat is either:

1. Combined with oxygen to create energy, water, and carbon dioxide.

- OR –

2. Used to make lipoproteins: a group of soluble proteins that transport fat through blood plasma.

When your body utilizes stored fat, the process is still very much the same. An enzyme within the fat cells break down triglycerides (a type of fat that is stored in adipose tissue). This action releases glycerol and fatty acids into the bloodstream to combine with oxygen in order to create energy, water, and a waste product of carbon dioxide.

Carbohydrates

Carbohydrates are stored in small quantities because your body uses most of them for energy right away. This leads us to having short bursts of energy, followed by prolonged lulls of lethargy. The carbs we consume as food are broken down into small pieces as glucose so that they are easily absorbed through the walls of the small intestines. As glucose travels through your body, it enters the circulatory system, which causes your blood sugar levels to rise. When your cells have taken in as much glucose as they can, your liver stores most of the excess glucose to burn for energy between meals. This is when your blood sugar falls once again. If there is any leftover glucose still to be used, it is turned into fat for long-term storage. When your body does not receive carbohydrates for a significant amount of time, your body primarily functions off of stored fat by liquidating the fat tissue.

As previously mentioned, fat may be good for you but it is not calorie free whatsoever. Fat contains a high number of calories, which can be harmful to your weight loss goals when consumed in excess. Therefore, while your fat intake should be around seventy-percent of your macronutrients, you need to be careful of just how many calories you're consuming.

Even if you choose not to pay close attention to your calories or macros, it is beneficial to at least practice some control while consuming fats. You can do this by measuring your fats and oils before consuming them. For example, salad dressing that contains olive oil can quickly accumulate just by trying to "eyeball" the amount onto your salad. If you measure out the correct serving size, then you will be able to roughly keep track of your calories and fats so that you can stay on track with your health and fitness goals.

Chapter 3:
The Benefits of a Ketogenic Diet

There are many benefits to switching to a ketogenic diet, besides weight loss; and many of them are downright miraculous. Many people have reported life-changing results that have allowed them to become free of disease and able to live life to the fullest. One of the toughest parts about switching to a no carb diet is having to say 'no' to tempting foods and suffering from sugar cravings. However, even with the most severe sugar withdrawal symptoms, finally freeing yourself from the addiction of carbs and personally experiencing the effects of a ketogenic diet will make you confident in your decision to go no-carb. Here is a list of the most amazing proven benefits of changing to a ketogenic lifestyle.

1. Rapid Weight Loss

After years of trying every diet plan under the sun, you still may not have lost any real weight. Many studies, as well as years of personal experience from the millions of people who live a ketogenic lifestyle, have shown that you will achieve weight loss success on a low-carb, high-fat diet. The first type of weight loss you will experience is shedding water weight. Any water retention that you have will dissipate within the first few days of going keto; which will result in you losing between one to five pounds within the first week. Next, having depleted your glucose stores, your body will begin burning *pure fat* to convert to energy.

2. Your Blood Sugar Levels Will Improve

It has been shown through various studies that low carb diets will reduce the levels of glucose and glycated hemoglobin in your system. High blood sugar levels are common among individuals who have prediabetes, diabetes, and metabolic syndrome. When your body is constantly producing insulin in order to bring your blood sugar levels down, it eventually becomes unresponsive and insulin and leptin resistant. This results in type two diabetes; which has many severe symptoms including: excessive thirst and hunger, blurred vision, slow healing cuts and sores, fatigue, headaches, etc.

3. Your Blood Pressure Will Improve

High blood pressure is extremely dangerous and can result in miscarriage, stroke, heart disease, and heart attack. While it may sound counterintuitive to eat more fat when your blood pressure is already high, a low-carb, high-fat diet will actually improve your blood pressure and keep it low. A ketogenic diet is especially beneficial for individuals who are prone to heart disease, are overweight, or obese.

4. Your Triglycerides Will Improve

Blood levels with high triglycerides are a key risk factor for developing cardiovascular disease. High serum triglycerides are directly correlated with abnormal lipoprotein metabolism, obesity, diabetes, and lower HDL cholesterol levels. There have been various studies that have proven that a restricted carbohydrate diet lowers levels of triglycerides dramatically.

5. Your HDL Cholesterol Levels Will Improve

Just like being told that eating fat makes you fat, we have also been lead to believe that having high cholesterol is bad. However, there are two types of cholesterol that affect your health: HDL and LDL. High-Density Lipoprotein cholesterol (HDL) is good for you and helps your body function. Low HDL cholesterol levels is directly linked to coronary heart disease and other serious cardiovascular conditions that contribute to the mortality of both men and women. Not only will switching to a ketogenic diet reduce your risk of heart disease, but also improve your HDL cholesterol blood levels.

6. Your LDL Cholesterol Particle Size Will Improve

Low-Density Lipoprotein Cholesterol (LDL) accounts for most of your body's cholesterol. This type of cholesterol is regarded as bad for your health because having increased levels may lead to plaque buildup in the arteries, resulting in stroke or heart disease. LDL cholesterol particles come in different sizes: large, puffy molecules, and tiny, dense molecules. Scientific studies have shown that the density and size of LDL particles matter. An increased number of small, dense molecules has shown to hold a greater risk factor in the development of coronary heart disease. However, large, puffy LDL molecules can actually protect against heart disease. A carb restrictive diet positively affects the size of LDL molecules by eliminating the number of smaller particles.

7. Your Resistance to Insulin Will Be Reduced

Insulin resistance is common in those who have prediabetes, type two diabetes, obesity, and metabolic syndrome. Insulin resistance is when your body stops responding to the calls to produce insulin, which occurs when an individual regularly consumes too many carbohydrates. Think of it like the story "The Boy Who Cried Wolf;" after crying out that a wolf was near so many times, the villagers stopped responding to the boy's calls. There is a strong correlation between insulin resistance and cardiovascular disease. The risk of developing both of these conditions is significantly lowered when you stop consuming carbohydrates.

8. Your Body Will Become Less Dependent on Insulin

Your insulin levels spike every time you consume sugar, in response to your recently heightened blood sugar levels. For individuals with type two diabetes, their pancreases either do not produce enough insulin to efficiently lower their blood sugar or their body does not react properly to insulin. When your body does not have to constantly attempt to produce enough insulin to lower your blood sugar levels, your pancreas is able to heal and be conditioned to respond correctly when you do consume sugar. For individuals with type two diabetes, a ketogenic diet can in cases cure the condition and allow them to live life completely independent from insulin needs and blood sugar tests. High insulin levels are also an independent risk factor for heart disease. Lowering your insulin levels by switching to a keto diet will decrease your chances of developing a life- threatening condition.

9. A Ketogenic Diet Curbs Your Appetite

Eating sugar will only make you hungry for more sugar. Have you ever eaten so much food that you feel like you are about to explode, yet can hardly help yourself from taking another few bites anyway? Have you ever eaten a full meal, and not even an hour or so later, are already hungry or craving food once more? Everyone experiences cravings, especially when you are expending a lot of energy or are in the middle of your menstrual cycle. Hunger is the number one killer of a good, strong diet. However, studies have consistently shown that cutting out carbs and consuming more protein and fat has led to consuming *fewer* calories, experiencing fewer cravings, and feeling fuller for longer periods of time.

10. Most of Your Fat Loss Comes From Target Areas

Believe it or not, not all fat in your body is the same. Where it is stored plays a huge role in your health and risk of disease. There are two types of fat: subcutaneous fat and visceral fat. Subcutaneous fat lies underneath your skin, while visceral fat is held in the abdominal cavity, aka that stubborn muffin top that just won't go away. Visceral fat actually tends to form around your organs, which can result in inflammation, insulin resistance, and metabolic dysfunction. A low-carb, high fat diet can be miraculously effective in reducing the amount of damaging abdominal fat. Not only will you lose weight with a ketogenic diet, but you will specifically lose the most difficult fat to get rid of, which is nearly impossible to accomplish on any other diet plan.

11. Ketogenic Diets Have Therapeutic Effects for Some Brain Disorders

This benefit is almost too good to be true; and many modern medicine practitioners will tell you that it really is. However, low-carb, high-fat diets have been proven to improve, prevent, and even cure several brain disorders. It is true that your brain does need glucose; however, only a small part of your brain can use glucose, while the liver takes care of the rest. Your brain is also capable of burning ketones; which are created when your body is starved of carbohydrates and is relying on fat and protein to survive. The ketogenic diet has been used for decades to treat epilepsy in children, as well as improve the conditions of patients with Alzheimer's disease and Parkinson's disease.

12. Your Sleeping Patterns Will Improve and Insomnia Can Be Cured

Chronic sleep issues have become a major problem, especially in the United States of America. Nearly sixty million Americans each year suffer from some type of sleep disorder. What is possibly even worse is when you finally do get to sleep, but still wake up feeling tired and having to rely on high doses of caffeine to make it through the day. This isn't usually an issue until you actually have to go to sleep, in which case you are once again wide awake thanks to the caffeine. Does this sound familiar to you? Several scientific studies have shown that your sleeping patterns improve while eating a low-carb, high-fat diet. This results in more restful sleep and increased energy the next day.

13. Amazing Muscle Growth and Strength Gains

If you are looking to build muscle and become stronger with visible muscle definition, then a low-carb, high-fat diet is perfect for your health and fitness goals. The increase in protein will help your body build and restore muscle, while improving your recovery time. The increase in fat will also help to eliminate fat surrounding your muscles for better muscle definition, keep your joints working smoothly, fight inflammation, and increase the production of fat burning hormones, just to name a few improved functions.

14. Inflammation and Joint Stiffness and Pain Will Be Gone

C-Reactive Protein levels will indicate the amount of inflammation that you have. The key is to bring your C-Reactive Protein (CRP) below 1.0 for improved health and wellness. Inflammation can cause severe pain and discomfort, as well as affect your physical appearance. A ketogenic diet lowers your CRP levels naturally, reducing inflammation throughout your body. A low-carb, high-fat diet can also cure chronic illness and pain, including muscle and joint stiffness. Many people believe that getting older means learning to deal with terrible aches and pains, when it is possible to naturally control this discomfort just by eliminating sugar and grains from their diet.

15. You Can Fight Gum Disease and Tooth Decay

From a very young age we are led to believe that it is impossible to naturally cure our teeth from decay and rotting. Sugar that lies on your teeth and harvests bacteria is what causes cavities to form. After only just a few months of being on a ketogenic diet, you and your dentist will notice a change in the pH of your mouth, and the condition of your teeth and gums. In fact, any sign of gum disease whatsoever should have decreased after this period of time.

Chapter 4:
How to Maintain a Ketogenic State

Maintaining a specific dietary lifestyle for any length of time can be challenging, even for the most practiced athletes and dieters. However, maintaining a low-carb, high-fat diet for long-term success can present a number of challenges of its own: such as weight loss plateaus and anxiety about meeting your goals. There are however, thousands of people who have cut out carbs entirely from their diet and are truly happy with their results and lifestyle.

These tips will help you maintain your ketogenic state for a longer-term timeframe, as well as improve your own results so that you are always achieving maximum success with a keto lifestyle.

- Weight loss plateaus are very real, even on a no carb diet. Most people have no idea how to get past these periods of immobility and end up resorting back to their old eating habits. No matter how difficult it is to see the scale stay on the same number, you must keep strong in your ketogenic diet and continue to improve your willpower by fighting through the plateau. Your can do this by either cutting down on your calories even further for a few days, or by resetting your hormones by slightly increasing your carbohydrate intake for a brief period. It really depends on your body's individual reaction to each method to determine which course of action is right for you. But no matter what, don't give up!

- Start practicing intermittent fasting! Fasting has dozens of amazing benefit that have cured diseases, improved several life-threatening conditions, and promote dramatic weight loss. When you are finding it difficult to stay or enter into a ketogenic state, intermittent fasting may be the answer to your prayers. Intermittent fasting is when you do not consume anything except for water for a predetermined length of time. Fasting periods may range anywhere between eight to twenty hours, with only consuming water. Your method of intermittent fasting may change, depending on your goal at the time. For example, during a bulking or muscle-building phase, you might only fast between your first and final meals. But during a cleansing phase, your fast may last from your last meal to your first. This will help your body maintain a ketogenic state more easily, as well as to enter ketosis faster.

- Increase your sodium intake to fight cravings and improve electrolytes. During a ketogenic diet, you should consume three to five grams of sodium through natural foods: such as pink Himalayan salt or sea salt, consuming sea vegetables like kelp or seaweed, drinking organic broth, eating celery, or eating salted seeds or nuts.

- Always have a game plan for eating fast food. Sometimes we can't help but to be unprepared once in a while, and have to resort to eating fast food. It happens. However, just because you don't have a healthy meal already prepared doesn't mean that you can just surrender on your keto diet. There are ways to still eat keto while ordering fast food; such as asking for a burger without a bun, requesting for a lettuce wrap over a tortilla, eating a bowl from chipotle, or asking for extra lettuce and bacon on your burgers and then removing the bun yourself. Do not be caught unprepared in a fast food line.

- Always drink a lot of water to stay full and hydrated. It may seem like a no- brainer, but staying hydrated is not always an easy task. We often forget to drink water throughout the day, which leaves us feeling lethargic, tired, and stressed. Always keep a water bottle on hand, and try to drink at least three bottles of water before lunchtime, followed by another three to five bottles between lunch and bedtime.

- Remember that weight loss does not happen overnight, and there is no miracle cure to make it go faster or help you lose more weight. When we do not see results quickly, it is easy to get discouraged and give up altogether. It usually takes at least two consistent weeks of eating a pure ketogenic diet before you get into ketosis, for people who are new to it. Then, it can take at least another two weeks to start experiencing the full benefits of the keto lifestyle. Give your body time to adjust to this new diet, especially since it is so used to running on carbs instead of fat. Before you know it, you will be shedding fat and feeling more energized than ever before. Just believe in yourself and stick to your goals.

Chapter 5:
Breakfast Recipes

<u>Fried Eggs & Vegetables</u>

Ingredients:

- Coconut Oil

- Spinach (optional)

- Mix of Vegetables (carrots, cauliflower, broccoli, beans, etc.)

- Eggs

- Salt & Pepper

Instructions:

1. Add coconut oil to frying pan, and heat for 30 seconds

2. Add vegetables. If frozen, defrost in microwave first

3. Add eggs (2-3 eggs per person)

4. Add salt & pepper, or spice mix

5. Add spinach (optional)

6. Stir fry until ready

Bacon & Eggs

Ingredients:

- Bacon

- Eggs

Instructions:

1. Heat pan

2. Add bacon and fry to desired crispiness

3. Put bacon on a plate

4. Fry eggs in remaining bacon fat

5. Add salt, pepper, or seasoning (optional)

<u>Keto Pancakes</u>　(Makes 2 Pancakes)

Ingredients:

- 2 oz. Cream Cheese

- 2 Eggs

- ½ tsp Cinnamon

- 1 tbsp Coconut Flour

- ½ Packet of Stevia

Instructions:

1. Blend or beat all of the ingredients together until the mixture is a smooth consistency

2. Heat up non-stick pan with butter or coconut oil, on medium heat

3. Pour mixture into pan, and flip when bubbles appear

4. Top with butter, or a sugar-free maple syrup!

<u>Breakfast Tacos</u> (Serves 3)

Ingredients:

- 1 Cup of Shredded Mozzarella Cheese

- 6 Large Eggs

- 2 Tbsp. Butter

- 3 Strips of Bacon

- ½ an Avocado

- 1 oz. Shredded Cheddar Cheese

- Salt & Pepper

Instructions:

1. Cook bacon in the oven for 15-20 minutes at 375F.

2. Heat 1/3 cup of mozzarella on a pan at medium heat. (The cheese will become our taco shells)

3. After 2-3 minutes, slide a spatula under the cheese and drape it over a wooden spoon, resting on a pot (the cheese will droop over the spoon, creating a taco shape)

4. Cook your eggs in the butter in the frying pan. Stir occasionally and season with salt & pepper

5. Place eggs inside of your taco shells

6. Top with sliced avocado

7. Dice up bacon, and add to the top of the tacos

8. Sprinkle cheddar cheese on top, along with any additional seasonings or toppings you'd like!

Bacon Cheddar Chive Omelette

Ingredients:

- 2 Slices Bacon, Pre-Cooked

- 1 tsp. Bacon Fat

- 2 Large Eggs, Beaten

- 1 oz. Cheddar Cheese

- 2 Stalks of Chives

- Salt & Pepper

Instructions:

1. Heat a pan on medium heat with bacon fat in it

2. Add the eggs, chives, salt & pepper

3. Once the edges start to set, add bacon to the center and cook for an additional 30 seconds

4. Turn heat off the stove

5. Add cheese to the top of the bacon

6. Fold the egg over the top of the bacon to form a wrap shape

7. Serve with extra cheese on top

<u>Peanut Butter Pancakes</u> (Serves 2)

Ingredients:

- 4 Tbsp. Heavy Cream

- 4 Tbsp. Golden Flaxseed

- 2 Large Eggs

- 2 Tbsp. Peanut Butter

- 2 Tbsp. Maple Syrup

- ½ Tsp. Baking Powder

- 1 Tbsp. Butter

Instructions:

1. Mix together peanut butter, maple syrup, and eggs in a bowl

2. Add cream once mixture starts becoming smooth

3. Mix the cream in, then add flaxseed, and baking powder. Mix everything together

4. Grease a pan with butter, and put on medium-low heat

5. Add your pancake batter, and cook on both sides until golden

6. Serve, and top with butter

Low-Carb Waffles   (Serves 2)

Ingredients:

- 2 Scoops Whey Protein Isolate Powder

- 2 Large Eggs (Separated)

- 2 Tbsp. Butter (Melted)

- 1 Pinch Pink Himalayan Salt

- 50 Grams Cacao Nibs (or sugar free chocolate chips)

- ½ Cup Sugar Free Maple Syrup

Instructions:

1. Whisk the egg whites until stiff peaks form

2. Combine the protein powder, egg yolks, and melted butter in a bowl and whisk. If the mixture is too thick, add water

3. Add cacao nibs, salt, and egg whites to the bowl, and mix everything together

4. Cook the batter in waffle maker

5. Serve with sugar-free maple syrup

Raspberry Chia Pudding (Serves 4)

Ingredients:

- 1 Cup Coconut Milk

- ½ Cup Water

- 1 Cup Raspberries

- ½ Cup Chia Seeds

- 2 Tsp. Vanilla Extract

Instructions:

1. Place coconut milk, water, and raspberries in a blender. Pulse until blended (leave a few raspberries to the side for topping)

2. Mix the chia seeds into the mixture, along with the vanilla extract

3. Leave overnight in the fridge

4. Spoon into serving glasses, and top with leftover raspberries

Radish & Cauliflower Hashbrowns (Serves 4)

Ingredients:

- 1Lb. Shredded Radishes

- 3 Cups Riced Cauliflower

- 3 Cloves Garlic (Minced)

- Salt & Pepper

- ½ Tsp. Smoked Paprika

- 3 Tbsp. Olive Oil

Instructions:

1. Combine radishes, cauliflower, salt & pepper (to taste), and paprika in a bowl. Mix until all ingredients are combined.

2. Heat olive oil in a large skillet on medium-high.

3. Spread the mixture in a thin layer across the entire skillet

4. Fry until the mixture is cooked through and crispy

<u>**Keto Cereal**</u> (Serves 1-2)

Ingredients:

- 4 Tbsp. Butter

- ½ Cup Shredded Coconut

- 2 Cups Almond Milk

- Sweetener (optional)

- 1/3 Cup Crushed Walnuts

- 1/3 Cup Toasted Flaxseeds

Instructions:

1. Melt butter in a pot, on medium heat.

2. Add nuts to the pot and keep stirring

3. Add in coconut and continue stirring

4. Add sweetener (optional)

5. Add almond milk

6. Turn off heat and stir for a few more seconds until the mixture is completely combined

7. Serve

Chapter 6:
Lunch & Dinner Recipes

<u>Zucchini Boats</u> (Serves 2)

Ingredients:

- 2 Large Zucchini

- 2 Tbsp. Butter

- 3 Oz. Cheddar Cheese, Shredded

- 1 Cup Broccoli

- 6 Oz. Shredded Chicken

- 2 Tbsp. Sour Cream

- 1 Stalk Green Onion

Instructions:

1. Preheat oven to 400F

2. Cut zucchini in half length wide, and scoop out the flesh (leave at about 1cm thick)

3. Pour 1tbsp. of melted butter into each zucchini boat, and place in the oven for 20 minutes

4. Cut up broccoli into bite sized pieces, and shred your pre-cooked chicken

5. Combine chicken and broccoli with sour cream. Add additional seasoning if desired

6. Once zucchini is cooked, remove from oven and add your filling mixture to the inside

7. Sprinkle cheddar cheese on top, and place back in oven for an additional 10 minutes

8. Garnish with chopped green onion, and serve

<u>Cheese & Bacon Hot Dogs</u> (Makes 6)

Ingredients:

- 6 Hot Dogs

- 12 Slices Bacon

- 2 Oz. Cheddar Cheese

- ½ Tsp. Garlic Powder

- ½ Tsp. Onion Powder

Instructions:

1. Pre-heat over to 400F

2. Make a slit along the entire length of the hot dogs

3. Cut cheese into rectangular blocks, and place inside of the hot dogs

4. Tightly wrap 1 slice of bacon around the hot dog

5. Wrap 2nd piece of bacon around the hot dog, slightly overlapping the first piece

6. Secure bacon in place with toothpicks

7. Set in the oven on a wire rack, and season with garlic powder and onion powder

8. Bake for 30-40 minutes, or until bacon is crispy

9. Serve with optional salad

<u>**Chicken Soup**</u> (Serves 1)

Ingredients:

- 1 ½ Cups Chicken Broth

- ½ Cube Chicken Bullion

- 1 Tbsp. Butter

- 2 Large Eggs

- 1 Tsp. Chili Garlic Paste

Instructions:

1. Heat a pan for 30 seconds on medium-high heat

2. Add chicken broth, bullion cube, and butter

3. Bring to a boil and stir everything together

4. Add chili garlic past, and stir again. Turn off the heat.

5. Beat the eggs in a separate container, and then pour them into the hot broth

6. Stir well, and let it rest for a couple of minutes

7. Serve

Portobello Pizzas (Makes 4)

Ingredients:

- 4 Large Portobello Mushrooms

- 1 Large Tomato

- 4 Oz. Mozzarella Cheese

- ¼ Cup Chopped Basil

- 6 Tbsp. Olive Oil

- 20 Slices Pepperoni

Instructions:

1. Scrape out innards of mushrooms

2. Rub the inside of mushrooms with 3 tbsp. olive oil in total

3. Broil mushrooms for 4-5 minutes on high

4. Flip the mushrooms over and rub again with remaining olive oil

5. Broil mushrooms and additional 3-4 minutes on other side

6. Thinly slice the tomato

7. Lay tomato and basil into each mushroom

8. Lay 5 slices of pepperoni onto each mushroom and top with cubed mozzarella

9. Broil again for 2-4 minutes, or until cheese is melted

10. Serve

48

Cumin Pork Chops (Serves 3)

Ingredients:

- 1 ½ Lb. Pork Chops

- ¼ Cup Golden Flaxseed

- 3 Tbsp. Coconut Oil

- 2 Tsp. Cumin

- 1 Tsp. Coriander

- 1 Tsp. Cardamom

- Salt, Pepper

Instructions:

1. Season both sides of pork chops with salt & pepper

2. Mix together flaxseed, cumin, coriander, and cardamom in a bowl

3. Dip the pork chops into the mixture, completely coating the pork chops

4. Heat coconut oil in a cast iron skillet on medium-high

5. Once hot, add your pork chops and fry them

6. Flip the pork chops, and lower the heat. Continue cooking until completely cooked through

7. Remove, and serve with vegetables or salad of your choice

<u>Keto Pizza</u> (Serves 1)

Ingredients:

Crust:

- 2 Large Eggs

- 2 Tbsp. Parmesan Cheese

- 1 Tbsp. Psyllium Husk Powder

- ½ Tsp. Italian Seasoning

- 2 Tsp. Coconut Oil

Topping:

- 1.5 Oz Mozzarella Cheese

- 3 Tbsp. Low Carb Tomato Sauce

- 1Tbsp. Freshly Chopped Basil

Instructions:

1. Measure out all dry ingredients into a bowl

2. Add eggs and blend everything together for about 30 seconds

3. Heat coconut oil in a pan over medium-high heat

4. Spoon mixture into the pan in a circle shape

5. Once edges look brown, flip the crust and cook for an additional 30-60 seconds

6. Spread tomato sauce over the crust

7. Add cheese, and put pizza into the oven to broil until cheese is melted

8. Add freshly chopped basil on top, and serve!

<u>Reverse Seared Ribeye Steak</u> (Serves 3)

Ingredients:

- 2 Medium Ribeye Steaks

- 3 Tbsp. Bacon Fat

- Salt, Pepper

Instructions:

1. Preheat oven to 250F

2. Put steaks on a wire rack, and season heavily with salt and pepper on both sides

3. Bake in the oven for 40-45 minutes

4. Let the steaks rest for a few minutes

5. Heat the bacon fat in a cast iron skillet, and get the pan very hot

6. Sear steaks in the skillet for 30-45 seconds on either side

7. Serve alongside salad or vegetables of your choice

Warm Broccoli Salad (Serves 8)

Ingredients:

- 12 Oz. Bag Broccoli Slaw

- 2 Tbsp. Coconut Oil

- 1 Tsp. Fresh Ginger, Grated

- ½ Tsp. Salt

- ¼ Tsp. Pepper

- ½ Cup Plain Goat Milk Yogurt

- ½ Tbsp. Sesame Seeds

Instructions:

1. Preheat coconut oil in a large skillet over medium-high heat

2. Place broccoli slaw into the skillet. Cover and cook for 7 minutes

3. Uncover, and stir in the ginger, salt, and pepper

4. Remove skillet from heat and add yogurt and sesame seeds

5. Serve

<u>**Cauliflower Mushroom Risotto**</u> (Serves 2)

Ingredients:

-   1 Tbsp. Olive Oil

-   2 Cloves Garlic

-   4 Medium Baby Bella Mushrooms

-   1 Cup Chicken Broth

-   2 Cups Cauliflower, Riced

-   ¼ Cup Heavy Cream

-   ¼ Cup Parmesan Cheese

-   1 Tsp. Tarragon

-   Salt & Pepper

Instructions:

1. Cook garlic and mushrooms in olive oil, in a pan over medium heat

2. When mushrooms start to shrivel, add chicken broth and cauliflower

3. Stir well

4. Lower the heat so the dish simmers. Cover up and let it steam for 5-7 minutes

5. Remove the cover for 5-10 minutes

6. Once there is no moisture at the bottom of the pan when stirred, add the heavy cream, parmesan, and spices

7. Stir until cheese is melted, and then serve!

<u>Keto Kebabs</u> (Serves 2)

Ingredients:

- 200 Grams Chicken Breast

- 2 Peppers

- Paprika

- 1 Tbsp. Olive Oil

- 1 Lemon

- 250 Grams Haloumi

- Salt & Pepper

Instructions:

1. Chop chicken breasts into cubes

2. Chop peppers into similar sized squares

3. Take a skewer and pierce a chicken cube, pushing it to the bottom of the skewer

4. Do the same with a pepper square, and repeat until the skewer is full

5. Repeat until all peppers and chicken have been used

6. Garnish kebabs with paprika and drizzle with olive oil and lemon juice

7. Preheat oven to 400F

8. Place oven tray with kebabs into the oven for 20 minutes

9. Cut halloumi into thick slices

10. Place halloumi on pan for 5 minutes or until both sides
    have brown marks

11. Serve kebabs with halloumi and and any vegetables or
    salad you wish!

Chapter 7:
Ketogenic Smoothies

The following smoothies all make for great snacks, and each contain less than 5 grams of carbs! Blend all ingredients together in a blender, or NutriBullet, and serve right away!

Peppermint Smoothie

Ingredients:

- 1 Cup Cashew Milk

- 1 Scoop Chocolate Protein Powder

- ¼ Tsp. Mint Extract

- Handful of Spinach

- Ice

<u>Peanut Butter Smoothie</u>

Ingredients:

- 1 Scoop Chocolate Protein Powder

- 1 Cup Water

- 1/3 Cup Heavy Cream

- 2 Ice Cubes

- 2 Tbsp. Peanut Butter

Strawberry Smoothie

Ingredients:

- 1 Cup Unsweetened Coconut Milk

- 5 Frozen Strawberries

- 2 Tbsp. Heavy Cream

- 1 Fresh Sage Leaf

- 1 Tbsp Sugar-Free Vanilla Syrup (can be replaced with a small amount of vanilla extract)

<u>Egg Cream Smoothie</u>

Ingredients:

- 2 Raw Eggs

- 2 Tbsp. Cream Cheese

- ¼ Cup Heavy Cream

- 1 Tbsp. Sugar-Free Vanilla Syrup (can be replaced with a small amount of vanilla extract)

- 3 Ice Cubes

Chocolate Orange Smoothie

Ingredients:

- 1 Cup Cashew Milk

- 1 Scoop Chocolate Whey Protein Powder

- 1/8 Tsp. Orange Extract

- 1 Handful of Spinach

- Ice

Strawberry Coconut Smoothie

Ingredients:

- 1 Cup Unsweetened Coconut Milk

- 5 Frozen Strawberries

- 4 Tbsp. Heavy Cream

- 2 Tbsp. Sugar-Free Vanilla Syrup (can be replaced with a small amount of vanilla extract)

Frappuccino

Ingredients:

- 1 Cup Old/Leftover Coffee

- 1/3 Cup Heavy Cream

- 6 Ice Cubes

- 1 Tsp. Vanilla Extract

- ¼ Tsp. Xantham Gum

- 2 Tbsp. Sugar-Free Caramel Syrup (Optional)

Chocolate Avocado Smoothie

Ingredients:

- 1 Can Full Fat Coconut Milk

- ½ a Ripe Avocado

- ¼ Cup Cacao Powder

- 1 Cup Frozen Cherries

- ¼ Tsp. Turmeric

- 5 Ice Cubes

<u>Chocolate Coconut Smoothie</u>

Ingredients:

-   1 Can Full Fat Coconut Milk

-   ¼ Cup of Cacao Powder (or nibs)

-   1 Ripe Avocado

-   ½ Cup Shredded Coconut

-   ¼ Tsp. Turmeric

-   5 Ice Cubes

Salted Caramel Smoothie

Ingredients:

- 1 Cup Unsweetened Cashew Milk

- 3 Tbsp. Heavy Cream

- 5 Ice Cubes

- 2 Tbsp. Sugar-Free Salted Caramel Syrup

- Pinch of Pumpkin Pie Spice

Conclusion

Thanks again for taking the time to read this book!

You should now have a good understanding of the ketogenic diet and all of its benefits. Try out some of the recipes, and give the ketogenic diet a go! It really has the potential to change your life!

If you enjoyed this book, please take the time to leave me a review on Amazon. I appreciate your honest feedback, and it really helps me to continue producing high quality books.